Essential Oils for Weight Loss

Lose Weight, Burn Fat and Be Full of Energy

Table of Content:

Introduction

Essential oils have been a recent trend among people whether celebrities or not who are interested in losing some weight. Weight loss is good whether for health purpose or the sake of good looks.

Essential oils are natural yet powerful. Also, they are easier to follow compared to diets that alter regular feeding style. The research on essential oils is ongoing with many exciting discoveries already made.

Apart from the fact that essential oils are effective for weight loss, they are also useful in achieving balanced emotions, appetite control as well as a good scent for your body.

In this book, you'll find a short discussion about how essential oils work, why they work, some essential oils and how to use them as well as some essential oils recipes that you can make from the comfort of your home. That's a major advantage of essential oils the ease of preparation.

This book also mentions how you can work essential oils into your bracelet and necklace using ceramic diffuser beads to hold the scent of your essential oil all day.

I wish you success on your journey to weight loss using essential oils.

Chapter 1 – Why Essential Oils work

Different cultures from various parts of the world have known about the benefits essential oils have some of which are therapeutic and can heal. The abilities of the essential oil have been in full use for over 6000 years some to countries and empires like the Greeks, Chinese, Romans, Indians and so much more.

The essential oils are from various parts on a plant or tree. There are essential oils that they extract from the root, stem, bark, flowers and fruits. And for this reason, the essential oils in themselves will have different features that distinguish them from others.

A good example will be the essential oils that are known to have strong anti-inflammation properties, while others can be insecticidal or anti-microbial. In this light, there are also some essential oils that fat burning capabilities or help to curb cravings or unnecessary appetite.

How Essential Oils Work For Weight Loss

Your brain contains parts that are responsible for putting your body in the best physical shape and the right mental state, such that the when you stimulate these parts of the brain properly there are some have a general positive on you as an individual and this practice is known as *Aromatherapy*.

The human nose contains receptors that can perceive trillions of different kinds of smell, and they also have a crucial function of communicating to the amygdala and hippocampus in the brain, which are essential places where you keep memories and information.

Now for every inhalation of essential oils, study suggests that the amygdala and hippocampus are greatly affected such that they, in turn, influence our emotional and physical states almost instantly and directly, some of which are our motivation, mood, stress and sleep.

Even though presently there is no substitute for a healthy diet and regular exercising to help with weight loss, essential oils can go a long way to help with your weight loss target.

So eventually whether or not you fight a constant battle with cravings, low moods, slow metabolism, fatigue and emotional eating, essential oils can be that missing ingredient you need to achieve your weight loss target.

Chapter 2 – How to Use Oil Essentials for Weight Loss

Research by the Smell and Taste Treatment along with the Research Institute of Chicago resonated around the fact that continually inhaling culinary smell throughout the day (3-6 times)can go a long way in suppressing the desire to eat or taste anything especially when hungry.

Furthermore, the research advised that you should continue to change the essential oil you use across the day as this will help you to avoid the problem of familiarity with the essential oil, this will also bring a higher degree of efficiency.Here are some essential oils that can help you lose weight

Types of Essential Oil and How to Use Them

Cinnamon Essential Oil

It won't be strange to find that most people with diabetes use this oil.

A study done in 2013 indicated that cinnamon "has anti-parasitic, anti-oxidant, anti-microbial and free radical scavenging properties".And also that it tends to reduce serum cholesterol and blood glucose.

The study also indicates that cinnamon oil has excellent abilities in stabilizing blood glucose level and Glucose Tolerance Factor (GTF) in the body, this is essential because blood sugar levels could also lead to over-eating, lower energy levels, weight gain, sugar craving and even irritability.

By adding cinnamon oil to food, it can help in slowing down the rate by which glucose flows into your bloodstream, and this will help you in achieving your weight goals in the long run.

Cinnamon leaf oil contains eugenol, and this alters the neurosensory perceptions and also affect the way we taste and smell food, and this will help to reduce food craving and also stop overeating.

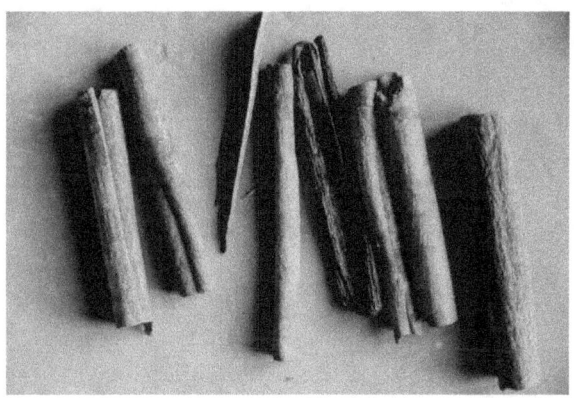

Using Cinnamon Essential Oil for Weight Loss:

- By drinking it: the FDA recommends that the cinnamon oil is safe to take directly internally, but it is advisable that you buy therapeutic-grade cinnamon essential oil.Therapeutic-grade cinnamon essential oil is 100% pure and toxin and addictive free.

  Therapeutic-grade cinnamon essential oil is unfiltered and undiluted. You can also add 1 to 2 drops of cinnamon oil into warm water (about a teacup) with a little touch of honey (raw honey would work fine and better) to help in the fat loss.

If you do this daily, it helps in reducing cravings. To curb late night food craving, it is advisable that have it before a meal or when the craving for food surfaces. You can also add cinnamon oil to your oats, baking or smoothies.

- Inhale directly: to prevent overeating before a meal or whenever a sudden carving sets in, you can inhale some cinnamon oil straight out of the bottle. As you do this regularly, it could go a great deal in improving your mood and make you fuller. It is advisable for emotional eaters.

- Apply topically: mix one to two drops of cinnamon oil with either of coconut oil or jojoba oil. After you do this, apply by rubbing it on your chest and wrist.

- Diffuse: put drops of cinnamon oil into your diffuser as this will not only give the house a great smell but will also help to stimulate a good mood.

Lemon Essential Oil

Lemon essential oils are known to be extracted from the lemon skin and containing the compound limonene, which makes lemon oil a characteristic fat dissolver.

A recent report recommended that when joined with grapefruit oil, lemon oil supported lipolysis (separating of body fats) making it a "suppression in body weight gain."

Lemon oil additionally detoxifies and take out poisons in the body that can be stored in the fat cells, slow down parasites in the intestines, and improve digestion.

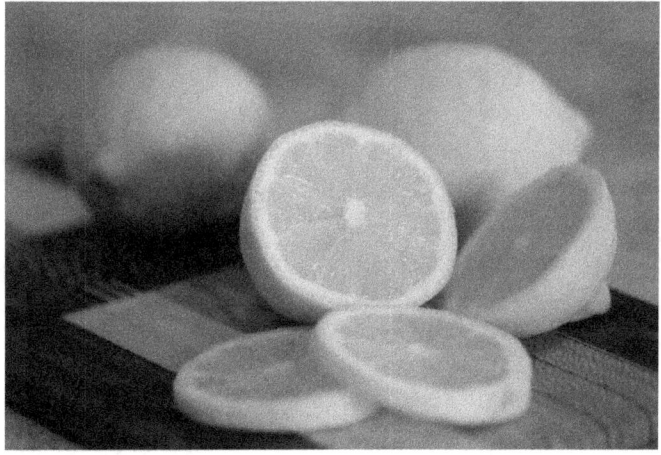

<u>Using Lemon Essential Oil for Weight Loss</u>

- Mix 2 drops of lemon oil to a glass of water in the morning and drink, this will help in detoxifying. It also supports digestion.

- Inhale the lemon directly from the bottle or soak cotton balls into the container and inhale directly from the cotton balls, this will curb cravings for food and decrease overeating.

- Blend the lemon oil with oils like coconut oil (carrier oil) and massage the mixture into areas that contain cellulite build-up.

Bergamot Essential Oil

Nervousness, gloom and low moods are frequently the major causes with regards to emotional eating

Giving in to your cravings may help light up your state of mind in the short term span yet over the long haul it just prompts sentiments of blame and low esteem, particularly when you heap on the pounds.

An ongoing 2015 investigation inferred that simply breathing in bergamot oil for 15 minutes can help your state of mind as well as decrease cortisol (a pressure hormone), that has a negative impact on fat loss.

In a recent report, 237 members with hyperlipemia (elevated amounts of fat in the blood) were given a fresh extract of bergamot orally for 30 days, and the investigation demonstrated that they could diminish blood cholesterol levels and altogether help in the reduction of blood glucose.

Bergamot contains polyphenols (a similar compound found in green tea), and it can push the body to dissolve fat and sugar normally. The sweet citrus aroma of bergamot oil gives you a high sense of feel, causing you to unwind and also smother cravings and control emotional eating.

Bergamot also has an enormous amount of limonene (additionally found in grapefruit oil and lemon oil), bergamot oil can burn fat. As indicated by University Health News, "D-limonene goes about as a gentle appetite suppressant and counteracts weight gain."

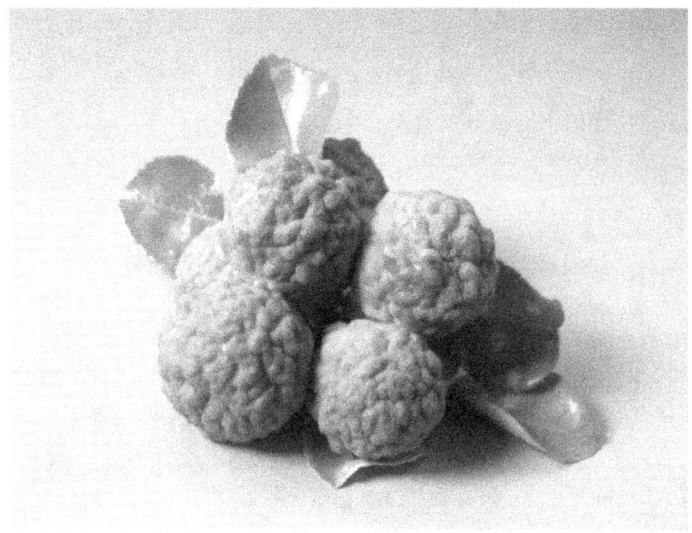

Using Bergamot Essential Oil for Weight Loss

- Inhale the oil directly or use a cotton ball soaked in oil, this scent of limonene will help to suppress cravings which in turn helps you to lose weight.

- Add this essential oil to your shower and cover the drain, inhale the scent to get the maximum benefits which keep you refreshed and in the right mind to lose weight.

Frankincense Essential Oil

Frankincense oil is gotten from the native of a tree local to Somalia, in Africa, and is fantastic for calming uneasiness and low inclinations that can trigger the need to eat more to food to feel satisfied.

Wealthy in sub-atomic structures called sesquiterpenes, that can cross the blood-cerebrum boundary, frankincense oil can ease the negative impacts of both uneasiness and misery.

Frankincense oil can encourage digestion by accelerating the flow rate of bile and gastric juices which in turn influences the metabolic rate and helps weight reduction

It can likewise stimulate peristaltic movement which enables food to move quickly through the digestive organs, improving digestion.

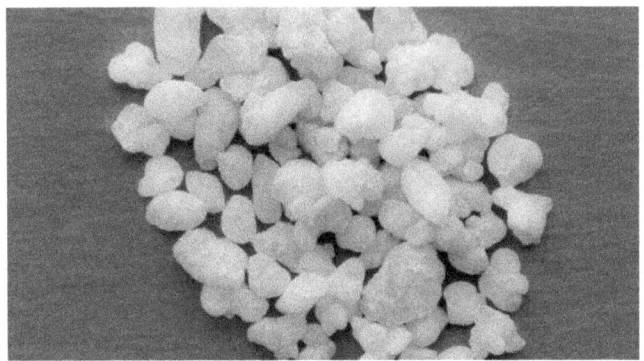

How to Use Frankincense Oil

- Inhaling a few deep breaths of frankincense essential oil will help subdue hunger pangs and induce a calm feeling.

- Add a few drops (2-3) frankincense oil to your diffuser and allow its sweet aroma fill the air surrounding you, this will help to lead away anxious feeling and calm your mind leaving you with lesser cravings.

Jasmine Essential Oil

Jasmine essential oil extracted from the sweet-smelling jasmine bloom, a research study recommends that the scent of Jasmine is very calming.

Jasmine oil has been utilized for quite a long time to cure uneasiness, low sex drive, sleep deprivation and misery; furthermore, research demonstrates that jasmine can calm despondency and elevate your mood.

This trait makes it a phenomenal fundamental oil to use if you are attempting to get in shape and can't control cravings and fell the need to turn to food when you're feeling low or experience difficulty sleeping off at night (which can prompt late night immense consuming of food).

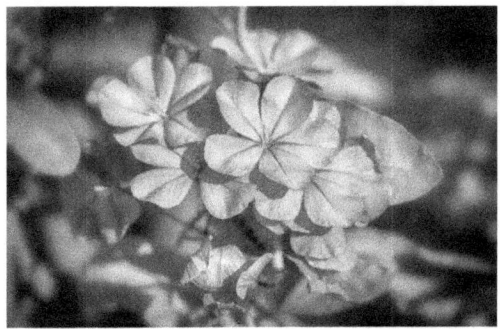

<u>Using Jasmine Essential Oil for Weight Reduction</u>

- Inhale jasmine essential oil before taking a meal, and it will help to calm your senses to prevent you from over-eating. You can also go further to put a few drops of this essential oil on your handkerchief and carry it along with you all day, inhaling from time to time.

- Combine about 2-3 drops of jasmine and about 4-5 drops of grapefruit oil in you diffuse which will send a citrusy scent that will keep you in a good mood and help relax the nerve that causes food cravings.

Orange Essential Oil

Orange oil can control appetite and reduce overeating. It contains Vitamin C and furthermore has a cancer prevention agent benefit. The sharp citrusy aroma is additionally a ground-breaking mood enhancer and can help many experiencing discouragements.

A research study from Japan's Mei University demonstrated that orange oil helped members decrease their energizer medicine consumption.

There are uncountable investigations which demonstrate that depression prompts weight increase and this one shows its direct relationship with really causing a higher hazard of obesity.

By utilizing essential oils like orange oil and different oils referenced above, you can lift your mood, feel much improved, and be less enticed to use food to feel better.

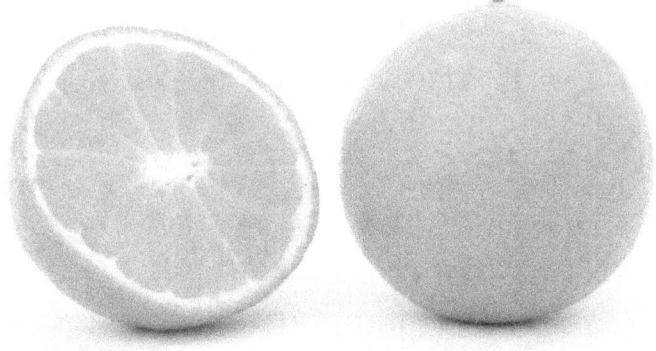

<u>Using Orange Essential Oil for Weight Reduction</u>

- Drink a glass of water containing 1-2 drops of orange oil before you take a meal to help reduce cravings and stop overeating

- Dab a cotton ball in few drops of oil and inhale directly to keep you perked up and stimulate your senses to keep you from overeating.

Rosemary Essential Oil

The rosemary essential oil originates from rosemary sprigs through steam refining. Rosemary essential oil is a solid, ground-breaking oil that can complete something significantly beyond flavor meat and potato dishes.

As indicated by a recent report directed in Japan, rosemary oil can diminish cortisol (the pressure hormone) levels in spit, and this is significant as high cortisol levels relate to dangerous health conditions, for example, hypertension and heart disease.

High cortisol levels lead to elevated feelings of anxiety, which can prompt emotional eating and weight gain. Keeping your cortisol levels low is critical to lessening your feelings of anxiety which will cause less emotional eating and keep your weight in charge.

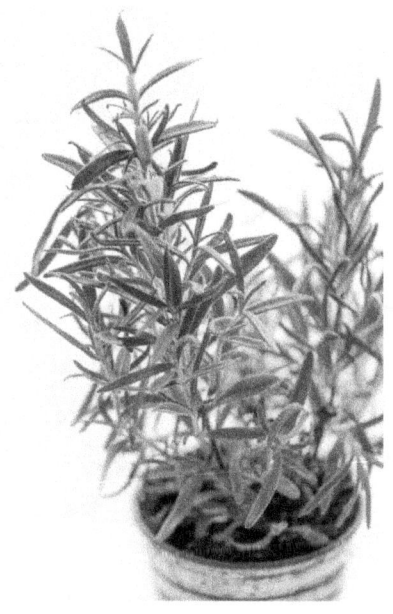

Using Rosemary Essential Oil for Weight Reduction

- When you feel stressed inhale rosemary oil for about 3-5 minutes taking as many deep breaths as you can help in reducing cortisol levels and help your waistline.

Grapefruit Essential Oil:

Grapefruit is well known for helping people lose weight for decades. The grapefruit diet also called the Hollywood Diet since the 1930s.

According to research, when mice are with food containing a lot of fat for three months, the mice were given grapefruit juice to drink gains up to 18% less weight than those that take water.

Grapefruit is gotten from the fresh rind, grapefruit essential oil is an excellent appetite suppressant, detoxifier and helps to prevent water retention in the body and to bloat as it also helps in dissolving fats.

It is a fact that the rind from which the oil originates contains a high concentration of nootkatone, which is a component which is responsible for activating AMP-activated protein kinase (AMPK). AMP-activated protein kinase makes the body reduce fat accumulation and use up sugar which in turn results to weight loss.

In a nutshell, AMP-activated protein kinase is stimulated by grapefruit oil which leads to more fats burned away.In another research, rats are also exposed to grapefruit essential oil 3 times weekly for fifteen minutes, and it led to reduced body weight and food intake in the rats

Limeone is another vital component of grapefruit oil that causes lipolysis (i.e. a process where the body dissolves proteins and fats), this allows reducing appetite and body fat.

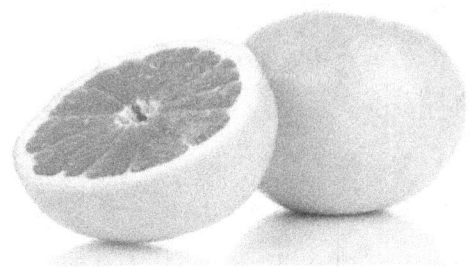

Using Grapefruit Essential Oil for Weight Loss

- Diffuse: put a few drops of grapefruit oil into your diffuser especially when you want to stop late night snacking.

- Dink it: put two drops of therapeutic-grade grapefruit essential oil in water, one glass full. You must ensure that you drink this every morning as soon as you wake up, this will help in increasing the reaction, detoxifying the body by flushing out toxins, increasing fat loss and helps in maintaining your weight.

  After taking a meal, you could also drink the grapefruit oil as it helps to digest food.

- Inhale directly: if suddenly, you are craving, the fresh scent of grapefruit oil can do a lot. You can decide to inhale it directly from a bottle, or you can also add a few drops into a cotton ball and inhale deeply. The scent of grapefruit makes the parasympathetic gastric nerve (the body mechanism that allows ghrelin-induced feeding) to relax.

- Apply topically: you could apply it by rubbing it on your wrist, temples, chest and also under your nose as it helps to curb appetite and also control carvings.

- Reduce cellulite: the oil is also effective in preventing water retention and also activates the lymphatic system. It contains a powerful anti-inflammatory enzyme called bromelain that allows and stimulates the breakdown of cellulite.

That is why many producers use grapefruit in many cellulite creams. If you want to reduce the cellulite naturally, try the chemical-free blend written below.

Grapefruits Essential Oil All Natural Cellulite Cream:

Ingredients:

15 drops grapefruit oil

Glass Jar

1/2 cup coconut oil

Instructions:

In a blender, blend the coconut oil with the grapefruit oil and store the mixture in a glass jar. Rub onto the part of the skin that has cellulite and massage for 5 minutes daily.

Ginger Essential Oil:

Ginger as an anti-inflammatory is necessary for weight loss as it reduces inflammation which allows a more efficient absorption and digestion of food nutrients.

In ginger, a compound called gingerols. Study indicates that this compound called gingerols reduces inflammation in the intestines and therefore makes the overall absorption of nutrients more efficient as it also helps in preventing diseases.

As long as your goal is to lose weight, the ginger essential oil will assist in absorbing the minerals and vitamins that you need to improve your cellular function and energy. You can be sure that it helps you to achieve your weight loss intentions.

A research done in 2013 showed us that ginger oil "possesses antioxidant activity as well as significant anti-inflammatory" properties and in about a month improved enzyme levels in the lab mice's blood had noticeably reduced chronic inflammation.

Another research in 2014 also indicated that to reduce obesity that is caused by increased fat diet, supplementing with ginger will help a great deal. The study also concluded that ginger is a "promising adjuvant therapy for the treatment of obesity."

Ginger oil helps a lot if you are having problems with fat belly. An article published in 2004 in the Biological Pharmaceutical Bulletin indicates that ginger is a cortisol suppressant.

Blood cortisol levels can be caused by High cortisol level which is also as a result of a hormonal imbalance and stressful lifestyle, and this could also push the body's natural metabolism out of place.

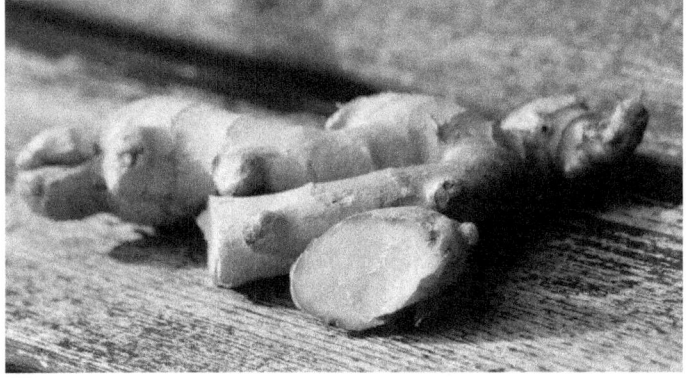

- By drinking it: FDA authorizes that ginger oil has no side effects or dangers when taken directly internally, but it is best and advisable that you use therapeutic-grade ginger oil for internal use. You can also include one to two drops of ginger oil into a warm glass of water and also a squeeze of lemon juice and some honey (raw honey would be advisable).

- Inhale directly: you can also inhale the smell of the ginger oil straight out of the bottle as it serves as a great pick-me-up and also reduces unnecessary appetites and food cravings.

Peppermint Essential Oil

Peppermint has been in use for quite a long time, and it has been used to treat indigestion and particularly when joined with caraway oil has it can help to loosen up stomach muscles and swelling.

The cooling therapeutic compound in peppermint oil, menthol, is phenomenal for improving digestion, expelling gas from the stomach and intestines and easing an irritated stomach.

Menthol can impact neurosensory discernments to change how we taste and smell nourishment, avoiding cravings for sugary sustenances, other sustenance cravings and curbing gorging.

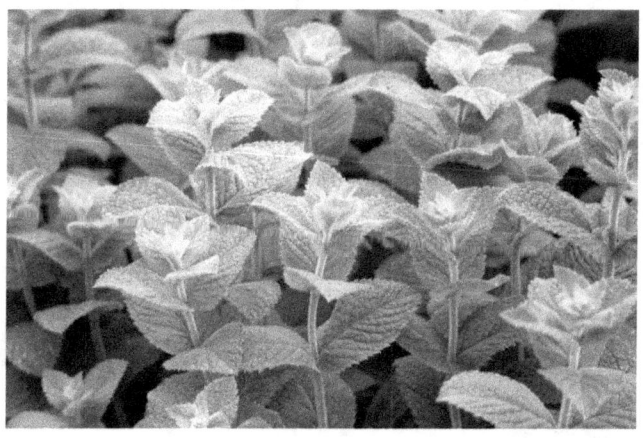

Using Peppermint Essential Oil for Weight Loss:

- Inhale it: You can decide to inhale it directly from a bottle, or you can also add a few drops into a cotton ball and inhale deeply.

The smell of the peppermint can take your mind away from food giving you a sense of relaxation. If you do this before eating, it can help prevent overeating and reduces your appetite.

According to the FDA, it is safe to take internally. About 1 to 2 drops of peppermint essential oil could also be added to a glass of water and taken before a meal as it helps to suppress and reduce appetite.

It is advisable that you buy and use therapeutic grade peppermint essential oil. Therapeutic grade peppermint essential oil is 100% pure and toxin and additives free. You can be rest assured that therapeutic grade peppermint essential oil is undiluted and unfiltered.

- Diffuse: by adding a few drops of peppermint essential oil into your diffuser especially when you feel like snacking. The mint scent is capable of curbing depression and will also go a long way in getting you energized.

Sandalwood Essential Oil

It is also advisable that you eat when you are stressed out if you are an emotional eater. Sandalwood essential oil also helps in reducing depression and creates a sense of calm. It has an exciting woody scent.

It also has a therapeutic effect on that part of the brain that dictates primal emotions like hunger, pleasure, anger and more. It makes a balance in your emotions, and thus food will not be something you turn to feel good. When this is done, you are a step closer to achieving your weight loss goal.

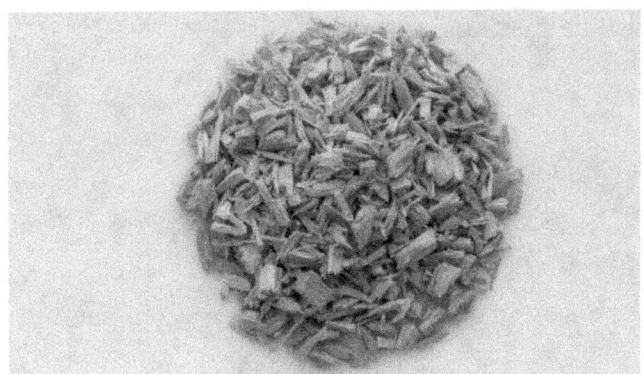

<u>Using Sandalwood Essential Oil for Weight Loss:</u>

- Inhale it: You can decide to inhale it directly from a bottle, or you can also add a few drops into a cotton ball and inhale deeply. The smell of the sandalwood can take your mind away from food giving you a sense of relaxation.

- Apply topically: you could apply it by rubbing it on your wrist and ankle as it helps to curb appetite and also control carvings after a long day's job.

- Diffuse: by adding a few drops of sandalwood essential oil into your diffuser especially when you feel like snacking.

Lavender Essential Oil

Each of the essential oils works in various ways in fighting weight loss. Some works in preventing fat accumulation, some others aids digestion, while others reduce appetite and lots more.

A significant factor that causes obesity today is anxiety and depression. "Feelings such as guilt, sadness, anger, and anxiety can often trigger series of overeating" says the National Centre for Eating Disorder.

Study indicates that stress and anxiety can be calmed by using lavender essential oil. Lavender oil also reduces that trigger that causes emotional eating.

Lavender oil also reduces cortisol level. Cortisols level has to do with the stress hormone that allows the body to retain fat which makes it tougher to lose weight.

A research done in 2010 by International Clinical Pharmacology indicates people using 80 mg per day of lavender showed less anxiety than those using a placebo. Another study done in 2013 shows that when rats are exposed to lavender for seven days inhibited depression-like behaviors and anxiety.

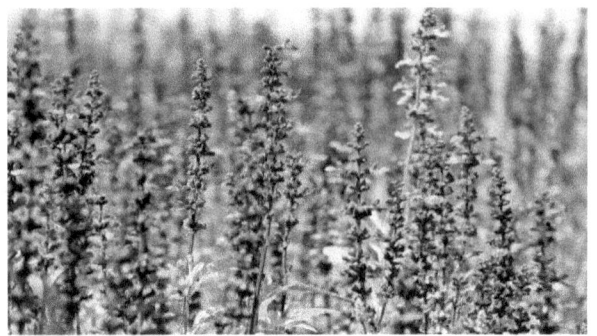

Using Lavender Essential Oil for Weight Loss:

- You can decide to inhale it directly from a bottle, or you can also add a few drops into a cotton ball and inhale deeply.

  The fresh scent enters the brain's center of emotion called amygdala and can take your mind away from food giving you a sense of relaxation and by adding a few drops of sandalwood essential oil into your diffuser especially when you feel like snacking.

  The pleasant aroma wafts around in the air and helps in reducing food temptation and anxiousness.

Chapter 3 – Essential Oil Recipes for Weight Loss

Weight Loss Capsule

Ingredients:

12 drops fractionated (liquid) coconut oil

2 drops lemon essential oil

2 drops peppermint essential oil

Vegetarian gel capsule (empty)

2 drops grapefruit essential oil

Instructions:

- ✓ Mix the coconut oil with the essential oils in a small container very well.

- ✓ Put the mixture into the capsule using an eyedropper.

- ✓ Use a capsule before breakfast daily to help with weight loss.

More recipes can be used at once to prepare capsule worth a week or even more.

Appetite – Curbing Diffuser Blend

Ingredients:

1 drop spearmint essential oil

3 drops grapefruit essential oil

1 drop ylang-ylang or rose essential oil

3 drops lemon essential oil

Instructions:

- ✓ Mix all the essentials oils in the ingredient list for this recipe in a diffuser.

- ✓ Before having a meal, diffuse one to two hours.

Essential Oil Boosted Drinking Water

Ingredients:

2 liters of drinking water

8 drops grapefruit essential oil

Instructions:

- ✓ Put the grapefruit essential oil into the 2 liters of water.

- ✓ To assist with the weight loss and also to eat less, take the 2 glasses of grapefruit mixed with water an hour or two hours before meal.

Weight Loss Foot Rub

Ingredients:

5 drops cypress essential oil

4 drops lavender essential oil

2 teaspoons carrier oil of choice (argan, avocado, coconut, sesame, sweet almond, jojoba, grapeseed, macadamia)

3 drops juniper essential oil

4 drops basil essential oil

8 drops grapefruit essential oil

Instructions:

- ✓ In a small beaker, mix all the ingredient above.

- ✓ Gently rub on the feet before going to bed (you could add water to increase efforts towards weight loss)

- ✓ You can use More quantity can be used for more than one use.

Weight Loss Massage Oil

Ingredients:

30 drops lemon ESSENTIAL OIL

40 drops grapefruit ESSENTIAL OIL

30 drops rose ESSENTIAL OIL

30 drops geranium ESSENTIAL OIL

1 ounce fractionated (liquid) coconut oil

Instructions:

- ✓ In a glass bottle, mix all of the ingredients above.

- ✓ Use it on your body taking your while taking bathing to help speed up weight loss, and you could use a professional massage session.

Citrus Anti-Cellulite Cream

Ingredients:

2 tablespoons witch hazel

10 drops lemon essential oil

30 drops grapefruit essential oil

¾ cup of coconut oil

2 tablespoons beeswax

Instructions:

- ✓ In a small bowl, mix the essential oils with the witch hazel.

- ✓ In a double boiler using medium heat, dissolve the beeswax and the coconut oil making sure that they melt.

- ✓ When you complete the above, remove from heat and mix the oils with witch hazel then stir gently to mix thoroughly.

- ✓ Put the result of the above step in a glass jar and wait to cool.

- ✓ Cover the glass tightly and store in a cool place. Wait for about 3 hours before making use.

Better Than a Tummy Tuck Cream

Ingredients:

15 drops geranium ESSENTIAL OIL

¼ cup beeswax (grated)

15 drops lavender ESSENTIAL OIL

15 drops grapefruit ESSENTIAL OIL

1 cup extra virgin olive oil

15 drops frankincense ESSENTIAL OIL

⅛ cup vitamin E oil

1 cup rose water

Instructions:

- ✓ In a double boiler, add all the ingredients above apart from the rose water and the essential oils.
- ✓ Place the mixture on medium heat until all the ingredients melt.
- ✓ Place the result into a blender and allow it to cool
- ✓ When you do this, blend the result until it is all thoroughly mixed (scrap the sides as you go).

- ✓ As you keep on blending, gently add the rose water to emulsify the mixture.

- ✓ Add also all the essential oil and blend quickly to incorporate them into the mixture.

- ✓ Add the cream into the glass jar and tightly cover it.

- ✓ Apply it daily on the abdomen to tighten the skin and reduce fat.

Chapter 4 – What to Look Out For When Buying Essential Oils?

It is vital that when you are buying essential oils, ensure that the bottle says '100% pure essential oil'. Also, make sure that the correct name of the species is well indicated in the label of the bottle.

If the word 'fragrance' is seen, have it in mind that there are almost always other additives.It is advisable that you buy essential oils from an organic source labelled as 'Therapeutic grade', this shows that they are toxin and additive free.

Therapeutic grades are undiluted and unfiltered. Be warned not to choose from Non-Genetically Modified Ingredients.

Conclusion

Closing Tips for Using Essential Oils to Achieve Your Weight Loss Goals

If you are a beginner to using essential oils, here are a few things that you should know to ease using them.

Firstly, it is advisable that if you are using essential oil as a newbie, ensure you do a body patch test on a small part of your skin (advisably your arm or leg) before you apply it on your whole body by rubbing or taking it directly internally. When you complete, whether you are allergic to an oil or not would be detected before you use a higher number of dosage.

Essential oils that pass this first quick skin patch test may be mildly irritating when you use them directly. You can also dilute your oil in a carrier oil like olive oil, coconut oil or jojoba oil before using it directly on your skin.

Ensure you limit the use of citrus-based oils (like orange and lemon essential oil) before using long period time outdoors, particularly during pool season and beach because they can be a cause of phototoxicity

Many oils are for external use only although it is not harmful if taken internally. But also make sure you get them fit for consumption before ingesting it.Lastly, always aim for the highest grade of essential oil that you can get.

Essential oils are implemented in various ways which are:

- ✓ capsules
- ✓ bath and body products
- ✓ massage oil
- ✓ diffusion
- ✓ rubs and balms
- ✓ inhalation
- ✓ food and drink recipes (when safe for internal use)

To achieve your weight loss goal, any of the recipes written above would apply. You can also take some recipes along with you to school, recreational activities, travel and work by making portable recipes. Your bracelet and necklace can be made with ceramic diffuser beads to hold the scent of your essential oil all day.

Essential oil isn't a miracle, they are only a push to your weight loss efforts. Don't stop your medication or prescription provided by your doctor. Using essential oil also shouldn't be a reason for living a reckless diet lifestyle.

Furthermore, problems such as depression, digestive disorder, autoimmune disorders, hypothyroidism and anxiety and other health and mood related issues associated with weight can be addressed using essential oils.

www.ingramcontent.com/pod-product-compliance
Lightning Source LLC
Chambersburg PA
CBHW070839310526
45788CB00018B/2608